This book is dedicated to my son and my beautiful, supportive wife. I can not wait to grow old (and strong) with you.

CONTENTS

Dedication

GO FIT YOURSELF Vol 1.   1

Chapter 1: Stop eating sugar   3

Chapter 2: Stop Drinking Alcohol   5

Chapter 3: Stop Consuming Seed and Vegetable Oils   7

Chapter 4: Eat Like This!   10

Chapter 5: Lift Heavy Things   16

Chapter 6: Check and Balance Your Hormones   21

Chapter 6: Get Quality Sleep   24

Chapter 7: Fast if You Feel Like It   29

Chapter 8: Celebrate Small Victories   31

Chapter 9: Keeping results for life   34

Chapter 10: Contacting Us   37

Books In This Series   39

GO FIT YOURSELF VOL 1.

Cut Through the Fitness BS

This is it, the last "diet" book you will ever need. I put diet in quotes there because it has become somewhat of a swear word. With today's fat acceptance movement changing the way we think about diets, no one wants to hear that word. I prefer the original latin meaning from Latin *diaeta* "prescribed way of life". While the world is moving away from the word diet and into "intuitive eating" or some other nonsense, the word diet simply meant a way of living. The word was coined before Doritos and diet soda, before seed and vegetable oils, and before desk jobs. It simply means, a way of LIVING to maximize your existence and time on Earth.

Now that I have that out of the way, I am going to introduce you, or reintroduce you, to the way you not only should eat, but the way you are DESIGNED to eat. I am going to skip quite a bit of the science because you are not here to read about all the studies I've read or anecdotal evidence that I have witnessed. You are here because you are sick and tired of being sick and tired, and I am going to give all the information necessary to live your best life NOT tomorrow, but today. Every chapter is going to have actionable steps and ways of making this way of life easier, because I'm not so ignorant as to believe you have all day to think about what goes in your mouth or what muscles you are going to train. Everyone has family, friends, kids, activities, and even brainwashing that will get in the way of this diet. I will help you stay the path no matter what comes your way.

CHAPTER 1: STOP EATING SUGAR

"Sugar is not good for anyone, at any time, with any goal." - Kyle Upton.

Yeah, I started this chapter with my own quote; sue me. I am going to take you back real quick to our distant ancestors. They did not have access to candy bars, soda, syrups, cookies, or granola bars. Heck, even just good old fashioned brown sugar was a luxury few would see in their lifetimes. IF you were lucky enough to stumble across a blueberry bush, the berries would be nothing like what we have cultivated today. It would be a small handful of sour pellets with larger seeds that you would save for quick energy to be utilized while hunting game (the real source of nutrition). Vegans did not exist, and even if they did, it was NOT by choice and they lived short, painful lives (I wonder if they still told EVERYONE in the tribe that they were vegan?).

My point is, not long ago in the grand scheme of things, no one consumed as much sugar in a month as almost everyone in the entire world eats daily. With this increased sugar consumption (particularly high fructose corn syrup, the world's cheapest way to make almost anything taste good) obesity has skyrocketed. A full 40% of the USA and Mexico is obese, with quite a few more overweight. Suddenly, having a healthy(ish) BMI is a rarity and puts you in the top 10% of everyone.

The problem is when I say sugar, you think sweet. This is not necessarily the case. If you ate a huge pile of rice or potatoes without any additional sweeteners, your blood sugar would spike like you just ate a candy bar. That is because almost all carbohydrates are converted, by your body, into glucose, a type of sugar you produce for quick energy. We as a species are bombarded by carbohydrates dozens of times a day from what we consume both in the physical sense, and ads that we are exposed to trying to make you crave the next carbohydrate hit. How often have you seen a fast-food ad and could not get the newest bacon cheeseburger iteration out of your head? The funny thing is, if you just removed the sugar laden, processed flour containing bun from the equation, you would have something resembling a healthy meal. But if you get the burger, the bun is essential, and you can't only have a burger, so you might as well get a side of potatoes boiled in vegetable oils (fries, duh). All of that was so salty, you might as well get a diet soda to wash it all down (diet soda IS healthier, all the doctors and dietitians say so). There is not a ton of added sugar in this meal, but your blood sugar will spike through the roof like you ate a dozen cookies.

Once again, science free, I am telling you: sugar and a large amount of carbohydrates WILL make you fatter. In large enough quantities over a long enough period of time, carbohydrates will help you develop type 2 diabetes. Carbohydrates will stop any of your fat loss goals in their tracks, they will make you a slave to hunger, and they will steal your motivation and cognitive abilities. These are facts, NOT just because I say so, but because they are true. Once again, sugar is not good for anyone, at any time, with any goal.

CHAPTER 2: STOP DRINKING ALCOHOL

This will be a much shorter chapter. I am 99% percent sure that everyone knows alcohol is not good for you. Alcohol of any kind, in any amount, will affect you negatively. Your liver takes a beating of course, but so does your brain, heart, and kidneys (you know, all the coolest organs). I know some folks that will say "the dose makes the poison" and to some extent that is true. If you would like to have 2 drinks twice a YEAR, the damage will be minimal and you can still muster up the courage to see your extended family on Thanksgiving. But if you follow the AHA's advice and drink 1-2 glasses of red wine a night for "heart health", you are doing your health and longevity a gargantuan disservice.

When you drink, almost all processes (fat loss, muscle building, brain repair, tissue repair, quality sleep) come to a screeching halt until your liver and kidneys can process and expel the POISON you have consumed. Depending on how much you drank or for how long, this will take a minimum of 24 hours, and sometimes all the way up to 48 hours! If you drink the recommended 1-2 glasses of red wine per night, or even just 3 days a week, you will very rarely, if ever, be in a fat burning or tissue repairing state. Basically, if you drink regularly enough, you WILL fall apart. It will take awhile, but your body will always be in a state of disrepair from which there is no coming back.

Despite the fact that I am a Christian, I am not a teetotaller. Part of my traditions for Thanksgiving and Christmas are having a couple of drinks composed of a high quality whiskey and some sparkling water. However, I do not kid myself that this is good for me, part of being human is sometimes doing things you like to do simply because you like to do them. I know that I am putting my brain and liver under stress, and I know that I will be 10 pounds heavier the next day. The point is, if you can't imagine a life WITHOUT alcohol, you need a therapist and AA. If you can have a couple of drinks a couple of times a year, go for it. Just know you are ingesting poison and putting the brakes on your physical (and maybe even mental or emotional) goals. If you are asking yourself "Well then what's the point of drinking?" The answer is there is no point and you can cut it out of your life immediately.

Quick and dirty tip: IF you use alcohol as an anxiety reliever or use it as a "social lubricant", look into kava kava. This plant, when made into a tincture and consumed before social functions, will make you feel more relaxed and easy going. It's like alcohol, but it isn't a total body poison and it won't lower your inhibitions (aka make you do dumb stuff).

CHAPTER 3: STOP CONSUMING SEED AND VEGETABLE OILS

Saturated fat and cholesterol are good for you, full stop. There, I said it. You have been lied to by "big vegetable oil" for many decades. Shortening, vegetable, canola, sunflower, and sesame seed oil are helping to keep you inflamed, to shorten your lifespan, and to keep (or make) you fat. For the following 2 chapters, I bet one of your thoughts was "but French people eat bread and pastries, they drink wine, they're breaking the first 2 rules and French people aren't fat!" First of all, French people ARE getting fatter like every other developing nation, just at a slower pace. Second of all, the reason they weren't getting fat for so long was because they don't cook all their delicious breads and pastries with vegetable oils. Instead of shortening and canola oil, the French still used real butter and lard, saturated fats that are nutritional powerhouses and anti-inflammatory.

I could talk about omega 6 fats to omega 3 fats ratio and how if the omega 6 fats are dominant in your diet, you are an inflammatory mess, but I will keep it simple and just say: Cook with and eat fats and oils that are as low as possible in POLYUNSATURATED fats. Vegetable oils are almost 100% polyunsaturated fat. These oils shouldn't even exist, vegetable oils are the byproduct of extreme processing, they are dirt cheap to manufacture and the profit margins are sky high. This is why they were pushed so hard in the fifties all the way to modern day. Crisco does not care if it makes you sick and fat, they only care that they are making a boatload of money off of chemical byproducts that they convinced you to put in your mouth. Every single fast food restaurant or gas station snack has a seed oil in it, or has been cooked in seed oils, once again because it increases profit margins, pure and simple. If you are at a sit down restaurant, ask them if your food is cooked in margarine or vegetable oil. If the answer is yes, make sure you tell them twice that you would like your food cooked in butter, lard, or coconut oil. If they cannot accommodate this request, leave and find a better restaurant, have enough self respect not to put your body through that meal.

More and more people are getting wise to the seed oil epidemic and its implication in the rise in obesity and premature death, and I could not be happier. INCREASE your consumption of saturated fats and ELIMINATE your use of seed oils and I GUARANTEE you will see noticeable improvements in body composition, energy levels and even hormonal health.

Cook with:
Duck fat (high heat sauteing and frying)
Avocado Oil (high heat sauteing and frying, avocado oil JUST barely makes the cut, use sparingly)
Ghee (clarified butter, high heat cooking)
Bacon Grease (medium heat cooking, food will taste like bacon, be careful)
Coconut Oil (medium-high heat cooking, food will taste like coconut)
Lard (baking and low heat cooking)
Tallow (rendered bovine fat, low-medium heat cooking)
Butter (baking and low heat cooking)

Eat/use cold:
Extra Virgin Olive Oil (most olive oil has been spiked with seed oils, check Google for pure brands)

Butter
The fat attached to your animal protein (untrimmed ribeye, the skin on your chicken, the yolk in your egg, etc.)

Never consume:
Vegetable Oil (seed oil)
Canola Oil (seed oil)
Margarine (seed oil that has been processed to be stable when warm)
Peanut Oil (seed oil AND a legume byproduct, yuck)
Sunflower Oil (seed oil)
Sesame Oil (seed oil)

The easiest rule I like to live by is this: Is it easy to extract the fat/oil from the source? If you have to go through 15 steps to get an oil, it is probably bad for you. To get coconut oil, you just need to squeeze some coconuts. To get canola oil, you need huge industrial machines and chemical reactions to create a "food like" product. I don't know about you, but I hate eating "food like" products.

CHAPTER 4: EAT LIKE THIS!

We've made it past the "don'ts". Let's get you eating a natural, human diet that will make you feel 20 years younger, get you to or help you maintain a reasonable weight, and increase your lifespan. It is the simplest diet you have probably ever tried, but it is not the easiest.

Before we begin, open your fridge, freezer and pantry. It is time to start throwing stuff away. Here's a secret: your "willpower" is a finite resource and it WILL run out! IF you have cookies and chips in your pantry, waffles and burritos in your freezer, and cheesecake and soda in your fridge; you will eat it eventually. Maybe not today, but at some point in the future you will come home hungry and stressed and eat that garbage. Throw away everything that is NOT an animal product, IS high in carbs, and DOES contain seed oils.

Now that we have thrown away the trash, it's time to restock. Meat and saturated fats of any and all kinds will be the backbone of the diet. Choose fattier cuts over leaner cuts. For example, chicken thighs with the skin on will always beat skinless chicken breast, both in nutrition and flavor. If you think you like chicken breast, try to eat it without seasoning of any kind. You will notice it is dry and disgusting because there is very little fat present. Now try that same experiment with the chicken thigh, skin on. It won't taste AMAZING, but it will be moist and flavorful all by itself, simply because of the fat present in the meat and skin.

Buy and eat with abandon:

Beef (filet mignon, ribeye, t bone, porterhouse, 80/20 ground beef. I realize the leaner cuts are usually less expensive and we aren't all made of money. If you can only afford chuck or bottom sirloin or other leaner cuts, drench it with olive oil or eat it with butter to increase the nutritional density, and 80/20 ground beef is usually as cheap as it gets, just don't drain the fat before eating)

Lamb (Chops, sirlions, untrimmed, whatever. It can be lean, so I usually just stick with beef, but there is nothing like a properly cooked rack of lamb)

Chicken, Turkey, Duck, Fowl (Dark meat and wings, skin on. the dark meat will be fattier and if you MUST eat the breast, eat it with the skin on or supplement by using 50% breast, 50% thigh WITH skin.)

Cheese (Full fat always, cheddar, mozzarella, cottage, bleu, feta, whatever. Avoid processed american cheese whenever possible, but I know it goes great on a burger and if it doesn't contain seed oils, I don't see much harm in it)

Raw Milk (Full fat unpasteurized only, cow, goat, llama, whatever. If you can not get raw milk, do not drink milk, insert legal stuff here.)

Eggs (Pasture raised and soy free if you can find them. Eggs are nature's multivitamin, if you can only afford the cheapest eggs, buy them, they are still better than NOT eating eggs at all. Obviously the best move is to get your own chickens, but I realize this can be difficult.)

Buy and eat often:

Bacon (Cook up a big batch and eat right away or refrigerate and use for snacks or as a salad topper. A wonderful blend of fat and protein, also delicious and filling, do not overcook)

Liver and other organs (I know, I know; not the tastiest, but probably THE most nutritious foods on the planet. If you can find a way to eat more liver, kidney, and heart, you will feel like a superhuman. Buy high-quality capsules as a supplement if you just CAN'T choke it down.)

Bone broth (Make your own and it is dirt cheap, if you are lazy like me, store bought is fine. Try to get BEEF, but chicken bone broth is fine too. Drink it once or twice a day or use for cooking and don't drain the juices. Wonderful for your joints, hair, skin, and nails)

Buy and eat every once in awhile:

Pork rinds (Not a great option, but high fat and 0 carb, use as a chip substitute if you are craving crunchy and salty, usually cooked with seed oils so be careful and use sparingly)

Beef jerky (Decent snack option, but often high sugar and low fat, check the nutrition label and ask yourself if it's worth it, often the only good snack in a gas station if you're desperate)

WHOLE fruit (NOT juice, whole pieces of fruit washed well with the fiber intact are acceptable, especially and almost exclusively before workouts. Don't overdo it, one apple or peach goes a long way. Also, bananas are sugar bombs, use sparingly.)

Protein powders (Whey protein and collagen peptides can be a great way to increase your protein intake over the day, especially during tough training cycles. The only issue is the lack of fat, try adding a teaspoon of coconut oil to your shake for a boost of saturated fats)

Sauerkraut, Kimchi, and Fridge Pickles (fermented, unpasteurized vegetables can be wonderful for your gut health. The bacteria that reside in your gut will use it as a snack and multiply, further increasing the amount of "good" bacteria while helping to fight the "bad" bacteria. Just a half cup of raw sauerkraut 2-3 times per week will help to balance gut bacteria, and it is pretty darn tasty with bratwurst. Check the ingredients, it should just be the vegetable and salt, NEVER pasteurized. The pasteurization process will kill all the bacteria in the food)

Primal Kitchen Condiments (while I don't recommend covering everything in various sauces, the Primal Kitchen brand of salad dressings, bbq sauces, mayo, and even ketchup will have no added sugar and are always made with avocado oil. The brand was launched by Mark Sisson, a man that truly believes in the ancestral lifestyle and fixing your health through food.)

Buy and use very sparingly:

Broccoli and Cauliflower (Broccoli and Cauliflower are delicious when cooked in butter and salt, a way to add food volume, and will help make wonderful bowel movements, eat once or twice a week if you want to, but vegetables aren't necessary in a human diet. NEVER EAT RAW, just think of these as a way to get more butter or cheese in your diet.)

Carrots (Organic and washed very well, same notes as broccoli and cauliflower)

Stevia sweetener (Use in place of sugar IF YOU MUST, but try to get away from "sweet" stuff, you are an adult and not everything has to be sweet, get the liquid version)

Lettuce (Almost 0 nutritional value, I use lettuce as a filler if I only have a small amount of meat OR as a way to get more fats using dressings, cheese, and bacon. Lettuces, and no other leafy greens, are simply a vehicle to get fats and protein into your body. Out of all the leafy greens, lettuce will do the least damage. Wash all lettuce very thoroughly, organic or not.)

Do Not Consume:

Leafy greens (kale, chard, mustard, it's all garbage full of poisons that the plant uses to protect itself against herbivores that might eat it.)

Legumes (peanuts and green beans are 2 examples of gut destroying, poison filled "foods" that no one should consume unless desperate or starving. Check the internet for the full list.)

Nuts (the risk to reward ratio for these admittedly delicious seeds concludes they are just not worth it.)

Most Other Vegetables (I am not anti-vegan or anything crazy like that, but vegetables will disrupt your gut microbiome and they contain various poisons used to protect themselves from animals that would like to eat them. Look up goitrogens, look up lectins, and look up foods that contain the most natural pesticides.)

Sugar (duh)

Grains (rice, pasta, flour, bread, pastries, cookies, wheat, seeds, it's all garbage)

Soy (soy has all the issues of vegetables, plus it is a hormone disruptor!)

Vegan Meat and Cheese Substitutes (these franken-foods are usually just soy, seed oils, and salt molded into the shape of actual food, they are not actual food.)

Lastly, I'm going to talk about "dirty" meat-based eating. While I would prefer that you get your fuel from whole food, minimally processed sources, sometimes life gets in the way. But eating low or no sugar, even from a fast food joint, would be better than eating buns or milkshakes. Here are some options. Remember this will be cooked in seed oils so do not get in the habit of eating fast food more than a couple of times per month.

1. Burger places (Mcdonalds, Culvers, Wendys, etc) - get a double bacon cheeseburger with a lettuce wrap, or on a plate with utensils. Add a 3-6 piece

chicken nuggets or strips for some extra protein.

2. Mexican places (Taco Bell, Taco Time, Chipotle) - get a bowl of whatever you want EXCEPT rice, beans, and chips. So you could get 2 steak tacos in a bowl with everything EXCEPT the rice or beans. Sour cream and guac can be great ways to add some extra fat and flavor.

3. Italian places (Olive Garden, Spaghetti Factory, etc.) - get a side of meatballs and italian sausage with red or white sauce and extra cheese. Or maybe a lightly breaded chicken parmesan with olive oil on the side for dipping. Load up on salad w/ a vinaigrette that contains only real Olive Oil and vinegar, and no soup or bread.

4. Asian places - Get the main course (chicken, beef, pork, whatever), make sure it's light or no breading and light sauce or sauce on the side. Ask about soy and if it can be omitted. No rice or noodles.

In summation, because I don't want you to get lost in the weeds, here is the quick and dirty of what you just read:

1. If it used to have a face, eat it.
2. High fat, medium protein, no or very low carb.
3. Minimally processed containing no seed oils.
4. A piece of fruit can be enjoyed as long as you eat the whole thing, no juicing.
5. Vegetables are mostly garbage and should be avoided whenever possible.

That's pretty much it, eat real food until you are satisfied, NOT stuffed to the gills, and you will change your life for the better.

CHAPTER 5: LIFT HEAVY THINGS

"No man has the right to be an amateur in the matter of physical training. It is a shame for a man to grow old without seeing the beauty and strength of which his body is capable."

— Socrates

This quote might be my all time favorite. Let me tell you: you were not built and put on this planet to be a lump on the couch, your office chair, or your bed. If you have no idea what a squat even is, but you are all caught up on the last season of "White Lotus", you are suffering. You may not know it but your muscles are in a state of atrophy and your metabolism is slowing down. You must get up and do what your body is meant to do: jump, sprint, walk, breathe, and lift heavy things with ease! I always tell my clients that strength is the base of the fitness pyramid. From strength flows power, endurance, balance, mobility, and the ability to live a fun life.

"Compound" movements, as opposed to "isolation" movements, are the name of the game. A good example is the standing barbell overhead press: The overhead press works your shoulders, triceps, abs, and even a little upper chest, making it a perfect upper body compound movement. Compare that to a tricep pushdown machine: The pushdown will work your triceps, and only your triceps, while taking balance, athleticism, and shoulders out of the equation. This is an isolation exercise. Also, it is a huge waste of time. If you can choose between a compound exercise and an isolation exercise, always choose compounds. We have things to do, kids to take care of, work to get back to, and people that are counting on us. We do not have time for isolation. Also, guess what will keep you moving longer and get you not only stronger legs, but a stronger body? If you said the squat, you nailed it. If you said the leg press, we have work to do.

Always choose the more "athletic" version of an exercise, even if it means you can't go quite as heavy or do quite as many reps. Stay on your feet whenever possible and do things that challenge your body as a "system", the way it was meant to work. Isolation exercises are for people with a lot of time on their hands, or people that just want to get a "pump". Your body DOES NOT work like that, your body is amazing, it wants to work your upper body vertical push, NOT just your triceps.

Good choice!	Waste of Time.
Standing dumbbell overhead press	Lateral Raise
Squat	Leg Extension
Deadlift	Leg curl
Dumbbell bench press	Cable flys
Chin up	Bicep curl
Bent over row	Rear delt machine
Push up	Chest machine
Power Snatch	Nothing even close
Kettlebell swing	Running

If you are unfamiliar with these movements, get a GOOD coach and learn them asap. These movements, when the load and reps are increased over time, will get you better results than any workout program you have ever tried. Every ounce of strength and muscle that you gain is another good month added to your lifespan. At the same time, if you can get your strength up, EVERYTHING gets easier. Running, jumping, getting up off the toilet, these actions are all effortless now, and you have officially solidified your INDEPENDENCE until the day your maker brings you home.

As an aside, here is what makes a good coach:

1. When you squat, they mention that you must stay in your hips, sit back, and don't be afraid to bend over if necessary for depth.
2. They are not heavy handed with praise, and always have a way of making you better at a lift. You know, "coaching".
3. They very rarely just put you on a machine and count reps.
4. When they are with you, they are zoned into you and your needs, not ogling a young lady doing hip thrusts or chatting with another member.
5. They are hungry for knowledge and always strive to get better at their craft.
6. They give you the knowledge to do it on your own, so that 6 months into training, he/she could cut you loose and you would know exactly what to do.

There is no shame in starting with bodyweight on almost all of these exercises. When I tell folks they MUST get strong, all of a sudden visions of huge, scary barbell movements start running through their heads. All I ask is that you get strongER than you were last week or last month. Coaching a 75 year old to their first below parallel bodyweight squat is just as gratifying as coaching a 200 lb high school linebacker to his first 500 lb below parallel squat. Start where YOU are, and slowly add weight until you are stronger, it is just that simple.

Absolute beginner workout program:

For the first week, I just want you to walk on a treadmill, any speed, set at a 2 degree incline for 45 minutes three times a week (Mon, Wed, Fri, or Tues, Thur, Sat). While you are walking, focus on staying just barely out of breath, to where it would be tough to hold a conversation. Do not run or jog, because running is bad for your knees and hips. Just throw on your favorite show or podcast and WALK.

For week 2, I want you to get a gym membership. Perform this workout in a quiet corner or with a trainer three times per week (Mon, Wed, Fri, or Tues, Thur, Sat)

1. Bodyweight squat BELOW PARALLEL (hip crease JUST below knee cap) - 2 sets of 5-15 reps
2. Push ups (from your knees or off an elevated surface is fine, elbows tucked, straight line from ankles to shoulders at all times) - 2 sets of 3-10 reps
3. Lat pulldown machine or assisted chin up machine or band assisted chin up (increase weight each time you use it by 5 lbs, start light) - 2 sets of 5-15 reps
4. Forearm plank (start from an elevated surface if getting to the floor is too hard right now) 2 sets of 15-60 seconds

Week 3-8, let's get you strong and independent. We built the base with the bodyweight movements, now we can incorporate weights. This is where a coach would be the most beneficial.

1. Barbell back squat - 2-3 sets of 5-8 reps (add 2-5 lbs each workout)
2. Dumbbell overhead press - 2-3 sets of 5-8 reps (add weight once you get 2 sets of 8)
3. Barbell deadlift - 2 sets, 1 set heavy of 5 reps, 1 set light with 20% less weight for 6-10 reps (Increase weight of the heavy set by 5 lbs each workout)
4. Assisted chin up machine or lat pulldown machine

- 2 sets of 5 reps (Increase weight 5 lbs per workout)
5. Push ups - 1 set of ASMAP (as many as possible), until you hit 20 unbroken reps, then elevate feet.
6. Seated horizontal row or bent over row - 1 set matching your pushups, trying to get close to failure around 10-20 reps.

Just because we have less time for walking does not mean I want you to stop. You can walk for 10-20 minutes after your strength workout, or break it up into 5 minutes walking before your workout and 10 minutes walking after your workout. On your off days, I want you to get AT LEAST 6000 steps. You don't have to do it at the gym, just keep moving, remember you were made to move and have fun, not be a lump on the couch!

For way more workouts and programs for everyone novice to advanced, buy my other book specifically focused on training.

Cliffs notes
1. You were not made to be a bump on the couch
2. Lift heavy things (with a good coach if possible)
3. Strength is the gateway to everything you want to accomplish in life
4. Start my absolute beginner workout today

CHAPTER 6: CHECK AND BALANCE YOUR HORMONES

Hormones make you who you are. Testosterone, estrogen, ghrelin, cortisol, these are the key players (usually) in how you feel, how you act towards others, and how effective your workouts will be. I know it can be expensive, but go to an endocrinologist and have your blood tested for everything. We don't care about your blood pressure or cholesterol levels (keep your triglyceride levels under control though), we are trying to see where your hormone levels are. Avoid high cortisol and elevated estrogen if you are a male, and watch out for high cortisol and elevated testosterone if you are a female. Tell them to check your thyroid as well, and get that balanced if necessary. If you have hypothyroidism, you will find it very difficult to lose weight and gain muscle. If you have hyperthyroidism, you will find it difficult to gain any kind of quality weight (or just sit still).

DO NOT go to your normal doctor and base your results on "average" testosterone levels. The average for men is anywhere from 250 total testosterone(!?) to around 700. This is the range at your normal doctor's office. An endocrinologist that knows what they are doing will recognize immediately that anything under 800 is a red flag. Also, keep a close eye on your "free" testosterone, this is testosterone that you can actually use. You want this number to be between 10-25 ng/dl (nanograms per deciliter) in order to feel your best if you are a man. If you are a woman, your free test should exist, but be more in the 1-3 ng/dl range.

Testosterone is what makes you feel "masculine". It increases your motivation, helps you deal with life, and of course builds muscle and burns fat. If you have low total and free testosterone levels, I guarantee if you get those up, you will feel like a new man. Try to increase levels naturally at first, and introduce exogenous testosterone as your "nuclear" option if nothing else works. The quickest way to get your testosterone up to it's natural limits is to increase your fatty red meat consumption, get 7.5-9 hours of sleep per night, and add at least 5,000 IUs of vitamin D3 + K2 to your supplement regimen. These are fat soluble vitamins, so take them with food that has fat in it. The reason saturated fat is so good at raising your testosterone is because it contains cholesterol. While cholesterol has gotten a bad rap, IT IS WHAT YOUR HORMONES ARE MADE OF. Think of cholesterol as undeveloped testosterone. If your doctor ever tells you that your cholesterol is high (even the "bad" cholesterol, which does not exist btw) and tries to put you on a statin, get a new doctor. The only part of cholesterol you should be worried about is your TRIGLYCERIDES. Take your triglyceride levels and divide them by your HDL levels, if the resulting number is less than or equal to 2, you are healthy as a horse (heart-wise). If the number is greater than 3, just exercise and sleep more and trust the diet to bring those levels down.

Estrogen is what makes you feel "feminine". If you are a woman and you are finding it hard to sleep, you are skipping periods for a reason you are unaware of, or you are feeling moodier than usual, you must get your hormones checked. Your testosterone and estrogen levels might be all out of whack and you wouldn't even know until you get them balanced and feel like a million bucks. If your estrogen is out of control or all over the place, eliminate all soy from your diet, eat more fatty meat, and increase sleep to 7.5-9 hours. Your goal should never be to completely eliminate estrogen obviously, but your hormones should be balanced. That means a low(er) level of estrogen in men, and a high(er) level of estrogen in women.

Cliffs notes:
1. Your hormones make you who you are
2. Get your hormone, vitamin, and thyroid levels checked by an endocrinologist
3. Do whatever you can to naturally balance these hormones
4. If all else fails, use exogenous (external) hormones

CHAPTER 6: GET QUALITY SLEEP

In the grand scheme of things, sleep is more important than food. There, I said it. You can water fast for up to 30 days (don't, but you could) without any big issues, but after 3 days without sleep you will almost literally lose your mind. Did you know that getting less than 6 hours of quality sleep per night is the equivalent to staying awake for 3 days straight, when testing for reaction times, alertness, and energy levels? My goal is to get you to 6 QUALITY hours of sleep per night MINIMUM. 7.5 hours is perfect, and 9 is acceptable if you are training especially hard or are simply exhausted all the time.

You will notice all the times I just gave you are in 90 minute intervals. That is because it takes about 90 minutes to go through a full REM (rapid eye movement) cycle. In the simplest terms, once you fall asleep you go through a "light sleep" phase of about 30-45 minutes, and a "deep sleep" phase of about 30-45 minutes. The deep sleep is where the magic happens. This is where your brain and muscles repair themselves, it's where you can rest psychologically, and usually it is where you dream. The issue is waking up in the middle of a REM cycle. Have you ever woken up wondering where you are and what year it is? You more than likely woke up during a deep portion of your REM cycle.

That is why a "power nap" is 20-30 minutes, which would have you awake before deep sleep. And a longer nap should be about 90 minutes (including 15 minutes just to fall asleep). Anything in between will have you waking up feeling groggy and asking yourself "what is the point of napping anyway?" So, aim for 15 minutes to fall asleep, and AT LEAST 6 hours of quality sleep, this will get you through 4 full rem cycles. Wake up at the end of a REM cycle and you will wake up feeling refreshed and ready to kick the day's butt! If you are still confused or refuse to do math, download the "Sleepytime" app on your smartphone or tablet and tap on "Go to bed now", it will automatically set an alarm for the end of a REM cycle. So whether you only have 3 hours to sleep, or you have 9 hours to sleep, it will make sure you wake up at the right time, just don't hit snooze!

Sleep environment checklist:

1. COOL, the ambient temperature in the room you wish to sleep in will be set to 65-68 degrees, you can use all the blankets and sheets you want, but your outside environment must be cool to get the deepest sleep.

2. DARK, get black out curtains for your windows and cover every inch. Turn your alarm clock on its face or cover the numbers with black duct tape. Get rid of EVERY external light source you can think of, even cover the tiny light on your TV (which shouldn't be in your bedroom by the way). IF you must have a nightlight for going to the bathroom or small children or whatever, make sure it is RED light and very dim. This will affect your circadian rhythm less than a white or blue light.

3. QUIET, when I say quiet, I mean no noises should penetrate your sleep. I understand we live in a modern world with sirens and dogs and HVAC units kicking on whenever, but you must do what you can to minimize their intrusiveness. Download an app on your phone that will play white noises (I like "Lightning Bug"), keep a fan running in the corner of the room, get a white noise machine, or have a friend make "whoosh" noises in your ear all night. The point is to have a low level, pleasant noise always going in the background to

prevent the sharper, stranger noises from rousing you from a deep sleep. IF that is not an option, you might think about complete silence using ear plugs. You will have to get used to them for a few days but if white noise is not an option, absolute silence is the next best thing. Do not leave a TV or radio on low, it is not the same thing due to the fact that the noise will always be changing (and you might have weird dreams).

4. No TV, smartphone, or tablets 60 minutes before bed. The blue light emitted from devices like these is a surefire way to mess up your circadian rhythms. Basically you are holding sun colored light about 2 feet from your face, making your brain think it is still daylight and preventing it from producing sleep hormones. Reading a book by red or very soft yellow light (man I miss incandescent bulbs) will not have the same effect, so if you need a light on before bed, use red or very soft yellow light bulbs. IF you MUST use your phone or tablet at night (maybe your hustle is online, I don't know), turn on a blue light filter. There are dozens to choose from, just put one on and use the darkest setting you can.

5. If you are an insomniac and you just can't seem to fix your sleep schedule even though you have tried all the tips above for a week or two, now we can bring chemicals into this.

WARNING: this protocol is habit forming, under no circumstances do this for more than 2 weeks and check with your doctor beforehand! Alright, that is out of the way. You will get yourself a small bottle of Benadryl or the generic version in TABLET form, not capsule. Then you will get a bottle of 1 MG sublingual (under the tongue) melatonin in tablet or liquid form. Last but not least you will get a bottle of ZMA (a mixture of zinc and magnesium that will relax your muscles). 60 minutes before snooze time you follow all the rules above AND take 2-3 ZMA (2 for female, 3 for male), ½ of a Benadryl tablet (just bite it in half), and ½ a MG of melatonin. Take this at the same time each night and after a few days you should be getting tired and falling asleep when and where you should. After you have a better sleep habit, stop taking everything except the ZMA. With this protocol, more does NOT equal better, do not increase the dosage on any of these items because you think it will be "more effective" try to fix your problem with the minimum effective dose, if it simply does not work in 2 weeks, stop the protocol altogether and join a local sleep study. To "fix" insomnia, go to sleep and wake up at the same time every single day. As soon as you wake up, jump out of bed and get some light in your eyes. Sunlight is the best, but ANY light will work in a pinch. We are simply trying to signal to your brain that it is day time and time to get up!

Wake up checklist:

1. FAST, wake up quickly, as soon as that alarm goes off tell yourself you have until the count of 5 to get up. Your feet must be on the floor by the time you say 5. This will prevent you from "snoozing" and waking up in a panic during a deep sleep cycle.

2. LIGHT, get light in your eyes as soon as possible. Once again, sunlight is your best option here, but I have used the bathroom light before if my wife is still sleeping and I need to get going. Don't stare directly at the sun obviously, just bathe in the light with minimal squinting for about 30-60 seconds.

3. SPLASH, throw some cold water on your face and neck to get the parasympathetic (fight or flight) nervous system excited for a bit, this will help get your energy levels up and increase your stress hormones slightly if you aren't going to workout.

4. WORKOUT, IF you workout at the start of the day,

this is the time to hit it. Wait until at least 30 minutes after you wake up. IF you don't workout in the morning, skip this step and get to work.

5. BREAKFAST, IF you just worked out, eat a good breakfast full of fats, a little protein, and no carbs. IF you did not just workout or you don't eat breakfast, skip this step. The point is to establish a routine where you wake up, eat, and workout at the same times of the day so your body knows when to release hormones that will help you conquer your day, and when to release hormones that help you wind down and get ready for a deep sleep.

Cliff Notes
1. Sleep is more important than food.
2. Quality sleep of 6 hours is the bare minimum.
3. Quality sleep of 7.5 hours is perfect
4. Sleep area is cool, quiet, and very dark.
5. Wake up quickly and get some light in your eyes.

CHAPTER 7: FAST IF YOU FEEL LIKE IT

My goodness I love fasting. I could go over all the benefits but it would take another book. Let's just say that what you have been told your entire life is a lie. That fasting is "starving yourself", that breakfast is "the most important meal of the day", that you need 4-6 meals to "keep your metabolism strong". Well I will tell you what, if you never ate breakfast again, you would be just fine, 4-6 meals are simply 4-6 insulin spikes to keep you on the sugar rollercoaster for life (and pad the food producers pockets), and that as long as you have body fat, it is EXTREMELY hard to starve.

The old 3 meal a day rule was made when people did not snack all day or eat heavily processed garbage full of seed oils. You would wake up at dawn, eat "breakfast" (literally "break-fast") around 6am, which would consist of a piece of homemade bread and a large serving of butter, plus a cup of coffee with some whole milk or cream. Lunch would be around noon with no snacks in between, consisting of a sandwich loaded up with meat and cheese on homemade bread, maybe some more coffee or water to drink. Dinner would be at 6 after dad got home, consisting of meat and potatoes. And that's it, maybe you would have dessert if your wife felt like cooking a pie, but after about 6:30, it's time to get ready for bed and you wouldn't eat until 6am the next day. So that is a 12 hour fast at night (including sleep), and about 5-6 hours between meals. This is the bare minimum that we should all strive for. If you are eating more than 3 meals a day, stop. It is unnecessary AND detrimental to your health.

Once you are off the sugar rollercoaster, you might notice that you don't get hungry anymore. That you don't get that 3 o'clock exhaustion anymore. Also that you are more level headed and deal with stress better. That is because you have transitioned to being a "fat burner". You are now supplementing your diet with your own body fat! In fact, when you wake up you might even feel like skipping breakfast. Well, this is me, giving you permission to skip meals. I guarantee nothing bad will happen to you, in fact only good things will come of it. You can skip breakfast, lunch or dinner and guess what? You will still be "eating" your own body fat! That is why you are no longer hungry, because you have become a fat burner, as opposed to a sugar burner.

Keep the fasts to around 16-24 hours and try not to fast before workout days (you will lose strength and explosiveness). In fact if you can plan to break your fast right after your workout, that is ideal to take advantage of muscle protein synthesis. Longer fasts can be beneficial for some things, but unnecessary for our goals of gaining or maintaining muscle mass while dropping body fat and living longer, better lives.

When you break your fast, get a good amount of fat and protein, and maybe some sauerkraut, pickles, or bone broth to replenish electrolytes. IF you eat a pile of carbs and seeds oils when you break your fast, I can almost guarantee you will be very hungry the next couple of days, maybe even fall back into old habits and backslide to the start of your journey. Of course, you never have to fast, you can still eat 3 meals a day and reap most of the benefits, I just needed a coach to give me permission to skip meals despite everyone telling me it was going to kill me. So this is me, your coach, giving you permission to fast. Only good things will come from it.

CHAPTER 8:
CELEBRATE SMALL VICTORIES

When people get started on a weight loss, muscle gain, or rehab journey, their eyes are always on the end goal. The problem is that the end goal is further away than they have been led to believe. In our world of INSTANT everything, instant dopamine hits from opening Instagram and liking family photos, virtually instant food served up hot from a fast food joint, and many, many programs offering "instant" results. If you need to lose 50 pounds of fat and you will lose an average of 1-2 pounds per week (usually less some weeks), your goal is at least 25 weeks away. It could take up to a year to lose all that body fat.

That is why I want you to celebrate the small victories. This will keep you motivated throughout your journey. At first, the only motivation you will need is seeing that scale number drop like a rock, but once that slows down or stops altogether, you will find it harder to stay the course. I would like you to weigh yourself on a digital scale with decimals included just once per week. Keep track of the number, if your weight goes down week to week (even just .2 lbs) or even just STAYS THE SAME, you are on track! If the scale doesn't move, I want you to be positive and say out loud "I am on the right track, I am no longer gaining weight". Then I want you to treat yourself, not to food of course, I want you to stop considering food the reward. Now the reward will be a deep tissue massage, or 15 minutes in the hot tub, or a shopping trip for clothes that you love and look great on you a size smaller than last month.

The point is, I want you to have internal AND external motivators. IF the scale weight doesn't budge for 3 weeks OR climbs back up, do not beat yourself up. I can not hammer this home enough, a bad week, or even a bad month, is no excuse to stop eating what you are supposed to eat and start back in with old habits. In fact, if you can have a week where the scale went up, but you are working on getting more sleep AND you hit all your workouts, THAT is a victory and I want you to celebrate it. The problem with your bathroom scale is that it can not differentiate between muscle and fat. If you ate a pile of salt the night before, you will be heavier, if you ate too many carbs, you will be heavier, if you are not getting any sleep and you are stressed to the max, you will be heavier. Have your coach take your measurements (especially around the waist, and I will bet you are losing inches (body fat), instead of losing scale weight.

One option for tracking small victories is something called an InBody, or EVolt scan. These machines will give you a pretty good idea of your body fat percentage. If you can get on one (look for them at supplement stores and good gyms), you want to see your "skeletal muscle mass" going up or staying the same, and your "body fat" slowly coming down (only use every 4 weeks, at the same time, and under the same circumstances). My favorite option for tracking small victories are PICTURES. Have someone you trust or use a mirror and take 2 photos, in your underwear, totally relaxed (do not flex or suck in). Take a progress photo every month and compare it to last month. You will be shocked at the progress you have made without even realizing it because you just see the same shape in the mirror day after day and it's hard to see small victories. This is my favorite tracking method, because who cares what an InBody says if YOU don't enjoy what YOU see in the mirror?

Cliffs notes:
1. Celebrate small victories with experiences, not food.
2. Just putting the work in IS a small victory.
3. If nothing changes for 2-3 weeks, check your sleep first, then what you are eating.
4. The only body fat test that truly matters is the old "eyeball" test. Do you like what you are seeing? Do YOU like how you are moving / how strong you have become?
5. Be patient, hitting big goals takes hitting a huge amount of small goals along the way.

CHAPTER 9: KEEPING RESULTS FOR LIFE

A gym goer asked me the other day, while I was going over my game plans: "When can I eat "normally" again? This is a question I get almost every time I get people off the sugar rollercoaster. First, let us define "normal" eating for 95% of the USA: Highly processed, highly palatable foods eaten in large quantities 4-6 times per day (gotta have those snacks to keep the blood sugar steady). They are really asking when they can have bread, pasta, beans, chips, sugar and flour back in their lives. The answer is never. I don't want to be TOO hyperbolic, but it is sort of like me asking people to stop eating arsenic and them asking when they can start poisoning themselves again.

The thing is, you don't want to eat "normally" ever again. Make a lower carbohydrate, meat based diet YOUR "new normal". Once you have hit your goal, you can relax a bit and VERY slowly increase your carbohydrate intake, in the form of whole fruit preferably, but raw dairy and fermented veggies could be an option as well. You want to find the carbohydrate intake that will prevent you from losing or gaining weight and stick to it for life. For most people, this will be between 60-100 carbs, depending on intensity of workouts and number of steps per day. But this is a guideline, the amount of carbohydrate you need to ingest to survive and even thrive is precisely zero grams per day, so start there and slowly work your way up.

IF you are celebrating something with food (Thanksgiving, Christmas, Anniversary, Birthday), I recommend going all out. If it's your anniversary or birthday, find a fancy restaurant near you and get the 4 course meal with dessert, try some foods that you haven't tried before and make sure the food is cooked with butter and quality ingredients. You don't want to stop your fat burning for Applebee's if you can help it. People often ask me: "You know Thanksgiving (or Christmas) is coming up, what do I do?" The answer is have fun! Eat the turkey, eat the sweet potatoes, eat the stuffing, it is one or two days per year where we can give thanks for the abundance around us and hang out with family and friends. I don't want you to be the weirdo asking for special food on the side or giving Nana a heart attack because you won't eat her mac and cheese. Just eat and drink whatever you want for a day, enjoy your family, and get right back on track the next day. You will be 10 pounds heavier due to salt, carbs, and booze if that's your thing, but you will have had a wonderful time and built memories with the people that matter most.

Always hit your workouts no matter what. I don't know where this quote came from, but it goes something like this: "Discipline takes over when motivation runs out." Remember earlier chapters where I said motivation is a finite resource? This is especially true when it comes to training. At first you are getting stronger and dropping body fat just with the walk from your car to the gym. Once it gets tougher, that is the true test. Are you DISCIPLINED enough to go to the gym even when you're exhausted, even when it's below zero and your bed feels really comfortable, or even when it's Thanksgiving? I keep a log book for my training, so I know what I did last time and what must be accomplished this time, and if a workout falls on my birthday, a major holiday, or a day where I just don't want to do anything, so be it. I will still go to the gym or take a hike because I know all it takes is 2-3 missed workouts and it will be THAT much harder to get going again. Here's a quick tip, if you are truly exhausted and can barely get the energy up to go to the gym. Just go anyway and walk for 20 minutes at a slight incline, stretch for 10 minutes, then just go home. The act of going to the gym means the chain is unbroken and you are ingraining that habit (just going to the gym) for life.

Cliff notes:

1. This way of eating is your "new normal" ; the standard American diet is no longer even an option.
2. For holidays, unless you have a binge eating disorder, just have fun! Eat and drink what you like and enjoy your family and friends.
3. Go to the gym when you're supposed to no matter what. Make it a part of your lifestyle.
4. Remember, have fun on holidays but get right back on your diet the next day, no matter what.
5. VERY SLOWLY add carbohydrates back into your diet in the form of raw milk, fruit, peeled sweet potatoes, or WHITE rice. Find the amount of carbs that will help you to MAINTAIN your weight for life, stick to that amount 95% of the time. Bread, beans, and pasta are still garbage.

CHAPTER 10: CONTACTING US

I know this stuff can be confusing, that is why I laid it out in very black and white terms. While shades of gray may surround our daily lives, this book is the foundation on which everything else is built. Read this book 10 times, or every day, I don't care. It is an easy, fun read that is great for quick motivation or to answer basic questions. However, if you have more questions or concerns go to these places for more info and in depth analysis of what I am getting at.

1. "Go Fit Yourself Podcast" wherever you get your podcasts
2. "Go Fit Yourself on Youtube"
3. Go.fit.yourself on Instagram
4. Go.fit.yourself on Facebook
5. A one on one phone call (30 minutes), is $50. DM me for details
6. Personal, one on one or small group coaching is $150 per hour, plus travel if necessary

BOOKS IN THIS SERIES

The Go Fit Yourself Series

The first 3 Volumes of Go Fit Yourself will cover nutrition, training, and lifestyle. Pick up all 3 to change your world forever, today.

Go Fit Yourself Vol 1. "Cutting Through The Fitness Bs"

In this volume you get an overview of nutrition principles so you can start eating (and sleeping) like you want to live a good life today!

Go Fit Yourself Vol 2. "How And Why We Train

In this volume I go over strength training and why everyone should engage in this particular form of fitness. Sample training plans included.

Go Fit Yourself Vol 3. "Living Like You Give A Damn"

This volume will cover lifestyle, mindset, and the Go Fit Yourself philosophies. It isn't Socrates, but it will get you motivated and off your butt!

For more information, check out The Go Fit Yourself Podcast on

Spotify, go.fit.yourself on Instagram, Go Fit Yourself on Youtube, or schedule a 30 minute phone call with Coach Kyle ($50, DM me for details).